Quick Reference Guide to Veterinary Radiography Kits

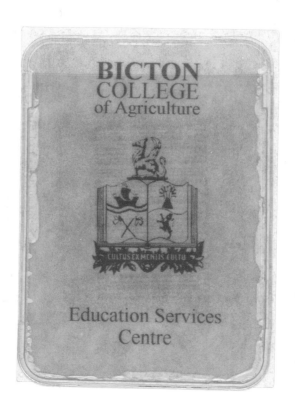

BICTON
COLLEGE
of Agriculture

CULTUS EX MENTIS CULTU

Education Services
Centre

Commissioning editor: Mary Seager
Development editor: Caroline Savage
Production controller: Anthony Read
Desk editor: Jackie Holding
Cover design: Alan Studholme

Quick Reference Guide to Veterinary Radiography Kits

Carole Bowden DipAVN (Surgical) VN and
Jo Masters VN

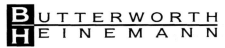

OXFORD   AMSTERDAM   BOSTON   LONDON   NEW YORK   PARIS
SAN DIEGO   SAN FRANCISCO   SINGAPORE   SYDNEY   TOKYO

BUTTERWORTH-HEINEMANN
An imprint of Elsevier Science Limited

First published 2002

ISBN 0 7506 4960 7

British Library Cataloguing in Publication Data
Bowden, Carole
    Quick reference guide to veterinary radiography kits
    1. Veterinary radiology – Equipment and supplies
    I. Title   II. Masters, Joanne
    636′.089′60757′0284

Library of Congress Cataloguing in Publication Data
A catalogue record for this book is available from the Library of Congress

Note
Medical knowledge is constantly changing. As new information becomes available,
changes in treatment, procedures, equipment and the use of drugs become necessary.
The authors and the publishers have taken care to ensure that the information given in
this text is accurate and up to date. However, readers are strongly advised to confirm
that the information, especially with regard to drug usage, complies with the latest
legislation and standards of practice.

Typeset by BC Typesetting, Keynsham, Bristol BS31 1NZ
Printed and bound in Great Britain by MPG Books Ltd, Bodmin, Cornwall

The
Publisher's
policy is to use
**paper manufactured
from sustainable forests**

II

Contents

Acknowledgements

The authors would like to express their thanks to Steve Dorrell of Veterinary X-rays for supplying a large number of the photographs for this book, Mr Alan Picken of BCF Technology for ultrasound images, Mr Michael Herrtage and Miss Jenny Smith both of Queens Veterinary School Hospital, University of Cambridge, for supplying additional photographs and images.

Introduction

The aim of this book is to provide an easy reference point for those veterinary staff involved in the preparation of radiographic procedures. It is not intended to be used as a textbook; more as a handy guide which can be kept in the radiography room for easy referral.

This guide will be invaluable to both student veterinary nurses preparing for a specific procedure for the first time, and to veterinary staff anticipating an unfamiliar radiographic procedure.

Each section is designed to cover the basic range of equipment necessary for routine radiographic procedures; however, flexibility for individual preferences should be assumed.

1
Radiographic terminology

Radiographic veterinary terms consist of two parts:

(i) THE PREFIX – or first syllable of the word; often used to describe the anatomy in question. For example:

arthro – joint
cyst – bladder
uro – urinary
gastro – GI tract

(ii) THE SUFFIX – or last syllable(s) of the word; often used to describe the procedure. Radiographical suffixes include:

GRAM – a recording, e.g.
Cystogram – a radiograph of the bladder
Urogram – a radiograph of the urinary system
Myelogram – a radiograph of the spinal cord

GRAPHY – method used to make a recording, e.g.
Cystography – radiography of the bladder
Urography – radiography of the urinary system
Myelography – radiography of the spinal cord

Radiographic projections

Cranial (Cr) – describes the neck, trunk and tail positioned towards the head from a given point. Also describes the aspects of the limbs proximal to the carpal and tarsal joints that face towards the head.

Dorsal (D) – describes the upper aspect of the head, neck, trunk and tail, and the aspects of the limbs distal to the carpal and tarsal joints that face towards the head.

Lateral (L) – describes the projection used when an X-ray beam is directed towards the left or right side of the body and emerges on the opposite side.

Lateromedial (LM) – describes when an X-ray beam enters a limb through the lateral side and exits on the medial side.

Mediolateral (ML) – describes when an X-ray beam enters a limb through the medial side and exits on the lateral side.

Palmar (Pa) – describes the caudal forelimb from the carpal joint distally.

Plantar (Pl) – describes the caudal hindlimb from the tarsal joint distally.

Rostral (R) – describes the parts of the head positioned toward the nares from a given point.

Ventral (V) – describes the lower aspects of the head, neck, trunk and tail. Towards the lower aspect of the animal.

Radiographic definitions

Cassette – a light proof covering for X-ray film, containing intensifying screens, in which film is placed during exposure.

Collimation – reduction of the beam size to the area under investigation – reduces scatter.

Contrast media – a radiolucent or radiopaque substance used to increase contrast within an organ or system.

Developer – chemical preparation that develops the latent image on an X-ray film.

Film Focal Distance (FFD) – an exposure value – the distance between the focal spot of the X-ray tube and the film.

Fixer – chemical preparation that fixes the developed image on an X-ray film.

Fluoroscopy – examination with a fluoroscope – continuous passage of X-rays that pass through the body and are projected onto a fluorescent screen.

Focal spot – small area where the primary beam needs to focus on the film.

Grid – a device made of a series of narrow lead strips used to reduce the amount of scattered radiation reaching the film and personnel.

Grid Factor – amount by which exposure time must be increased when using a grid.

Grid Ratio – the ratio between the height of the lead strips contained in a grid and the distance between them. Used to ascertain the grid factor.

Intensifying screens – screens containing calcium phosphor crystals which fluoresce, therefore reducing exposure time and intensifying the image.

Kilo volts (KV) – one thousand volts – measures the peak voltage used for an exposure time. Responsible for the penetration power of the X-ray beam.

Milliampere (mA) – the measure of the current during an exposure.

Milliampere seconds (mAs) – unit of exposure equal to the product of the mA and time in seconds.

Radiography – the making of film records (radiographs) by exposing film which is sensitive to X-rays.

Radiology – the science of using radiation energy in the diagnosis and treatment of disease.

Radiolucent – a substance that permits the passage of X-rays – appearing dark on the film.

Radiopaque – a substance which blocks the passage of X-rays – appearing light on the film.

Radiation Protection Adviser (RPA) – an external adviser (who has a specialist radiological qualification) appointed by the practice.

Radiation Protection Supervisor (RPS) – a supervisor appointed from within the practice, and who takes responsibility for radiation safety.

Scatter – scattered radiation occurs when X-rays are deviated or diffused by the substance they pass through.

Ultrasonography – an imaging technique used to view deep body structures recorded by measuring the reflections of ultrasonic waves which have been aimed at tissues.

2
Radiation protection

General health and safety

Ionizing radiation is used in veterinary practice for diagnostic radiography. As there is a lack of physical sensation and delay in onset of some of the tissue-damaging effects that can be caused by high doses or prolonged exposure to ionizing radiation, it is paramount that safety principles are addressed.

Three basic principles for protection include:

1 Radiography should only be undertaken where there is definite justification to do so
2 Exposure to personnel should be kept to a minimum
3 No dose limit is exceeded

Health and safety implications

Any veterinary practice using X-ray machines must inform the Health & Safety Executive (HSE) and comply with the Ionizing *Radiations Regulations 1999*. These regulations include the following requirements:

A Radiation Protection Adviser (RPA) will need to be appointed by the practice. The RPA will give advise on radiation protection, demarcate the controlled area in which it is safe to perform radiography and draw up a set of guidelines for *Local Rules* and *Systems of Work* relevant to the individual practice.

A Radiation Protection Supervisor (RPS) will need to be appointed within the practice. The RPS will be responsible for ensuring that radiography is performed safely and in accordance to the *Local Rules and Systems of Work* guidelines drawn up by the RPA.

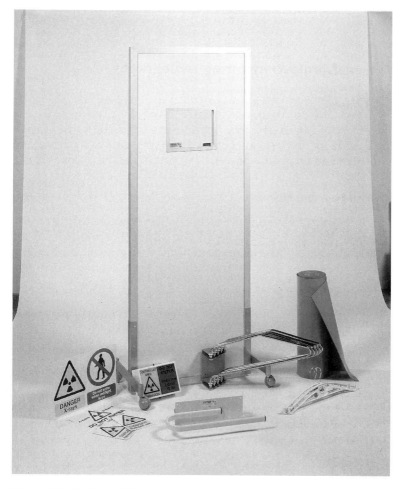

Figure 2.1. Health and Safety equipment – warning signs, mobile lead screen, lead protective sheeting, lead apron storage equipment (Courtesy of Steve Dorrell, Veterinary X-Rays).

Local Rules

Local Rules are instructions drawn up by the RPA which outline the details of radiographic equipment, procedures and restriction of access to the controlled area. The Local Rules also include a System of Work, which gives detailed step-by-step guidance to the necessary procedures to be employed during radiography.

Personal protection during radiography

Lead gowns

These should be worn by anyone present in the radiography room during exposure. Thyroid shields can also be made available for use.

Lead gloves and sleeves

These should be available for use when manual restraint is a necessity due to the severity of the patient's condition. Care should be taken to ensure that they do not fall within the primary beam.

Lead-lined table

The X-ray table should be lead lined to absorb any scatter radiation during exposure.

Lead screen

These mobile screens can be made available for any personnel who have to stay in the radiography room during exposure.

Dosemeters

Personal dosemeters should be worn by all personnel involved in radiography to record any radiation to which they are exposed.

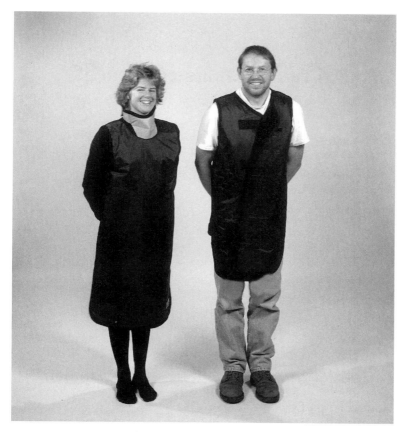

Figure 2.2.   Lead aprons (Courtesy of Steve Dorrell, Veterinary X-Rays).

Radiographic exposures

The intensifying screen and film combination chosen should be able to produce a diagnostic radiograph with the minimal exposure possible. Grids may also be employed to help absorb scatter radiation during exposure.

NB: During exposure all personnel need to be a minimum of 2 metres away from the primary beam and where possible out of the radiography room during exposure.

3
General radiographic equipment

The X-ray machine

Portable

- Easy to move around
- Commonly found in practice
- Low powered (20–60 mA)
- Longer exposure times needed

Mobile

- Difficult and cumbersome to move around
- Output power up to 300 mA

Fixed

- Stationary in the dedicated X-ray area
- Output power up to 1250 mA

The X-ray cassette

Purpose

A film-holder designed to house the X-ray film and intensifying screens in close contact.

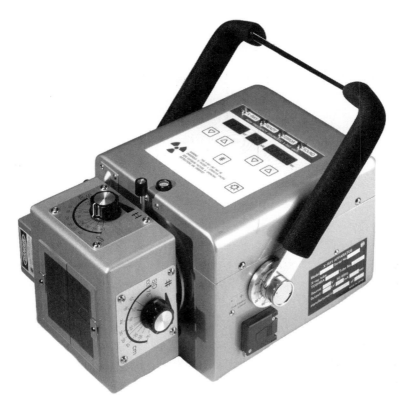

Figure 3.1. Mighty Atom 2 – output 60 mA (Courtesy of Steve Dorrell, Veterinary X-Rays).

Types

Firm
Commonly used in practice, older versions are manufactured from aluminium with more modern carbon fibre types being available in many practices today.

Flexible
An alternative to non-screen film. Plastic envelopes fitted with intensifying screens are used in areas where the use of a firm cassette is difficult, e.g. oral radiographs.

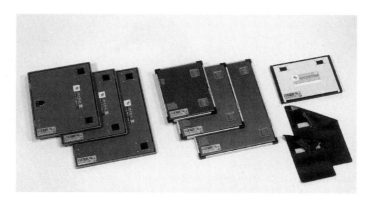

Figure 3.2. Firm cassette (right and middle: aluminium; top right: carbon fibre), and (bottom right) a flexible version (Courtesy of Steve Dorrell, Veterinary X-Rays).

Care of cassettes

- Keep clean – cover in plastic where there is danger of leakage from either patient or equipment
- Clean with soap and water monthly
- Number cassettes to enable easy identification of faults
- Take care not to drop

Intensifying screens

Purpose

Fluorescent plastic sheets placed inside the cassette between which the film is sandwiched. Mounted on the plastic are luminescent phosphate crystals which fluoresce when struck by the X-rays, thereby exposing the film. The light from the crystals is responsible for over 95 per cent of the exposure, reducing the amount of exposure to radiation required to produce a diagnostic radiograph.

Types

The phosphor used as the fluorescent crystal must emit sufficient light of the desired colour, and the size of the crystal will determine the speed of the screen. Larger crystals will result in a faster screen which has less detail, whilst smaller crystals will produce a slower screen with more detail.

Calcium tungstate

- Common in practice
- Fluoresces a blue light

Rare-earth

- More sensitive to X-rays
- Exposure factors can be reduced
- Finer image definition
- Fluoresces green/blue/ultraviolet light (film used must be compatible)

Care of screens

- Inspect for damage monthly
- Clean monthly with commercial screen cleaners and dry by leaving the cassette open in a vertical position

Films

Types

Screen film

- Made with silver crystals that are sensitive to the fluorescent light emitted from intensifying screens and X-rays; therefore requiring less exposure to X-rays
- The film must be compatible with the colour of light being emitted from the screen

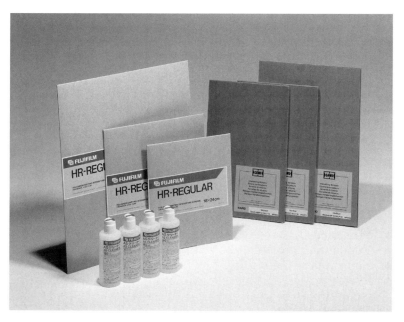

Figure 3.3. Intensifying screens. Green emitting on left, blue on right, with screen cleaner (Courtesy of Steve Dorrell, Veterinary X-Rays).

Non-screen film
- These films are not used with intensifying screens and rely on the direct action of the X-rays to become exposed; therefore greater exposure times are required
- Useful for areas where greater detail is required, such as oral radiography, as the use of intensifying screens does result in a loss of detail

Film speed

Film speed is measured by the amount of exposure required to produce a radiograph with good density.

- Fast film – larger crystals, requires less exposure but the final image lacks definition

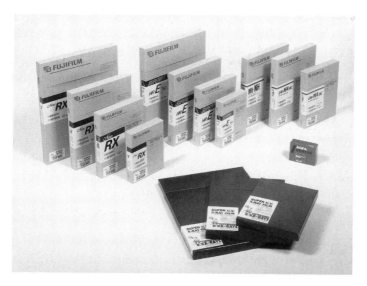

Figure 3.4. Film. Examples of blue sensitive, green sensitive, ultraviolet sensitive, and non-screen dental film (Courtesy of Steve Dorrell, Veterinary X-Rays).

- Medium film – most commonly used, compromise between exposure and speed
- Slow film – smaller crystals, greater exposure, greater definition

Storage of X-ray film

- keep in vertical position
- cool temperature
- away from radiation and chemicals

Grids

Purpose

A grid is designed to absorb scatter radiation and is placed between the patient and the film. It consists of strips of lead alternating with a material that allows the passage of X-rays. Scatter will be absorbed by the lead, thereby preventing 'fogging' on the film and improving the exposed image. The thicker the tissue to be radiographed (i.e. the density of the patient), the more the scatter which will be produced; therefore a grid is recommended for tissue thicknesses over 10 cm.

Stationary grids

These are either built into the cassette itself or are extra items of equipment which are placed over the cassette.

Parallel

- Vertical strips, parallel to one another
- May get 'grid cut off' towards the edges of the film due to the divergent nature of the X-ray beam.

Focused

- Central vertical strips which gradually slope away at the sides to prevent grid cut-off
- Must be placed the correct way up and positioned at the recommended film focal distance (FFD)

Pseudo-focused

- Vertical strips which are shorter towards the edges; therefore reducing the absorption of the primary beam
- Must be used at the correct FFD

Moving grids

The use of a grid which oscillates during the exposure preventing the visible lines seen on an exposed radiograph when using a stationary grid. An example is the 'Potter Bucky diaphragm' which is built into the X-ray table.

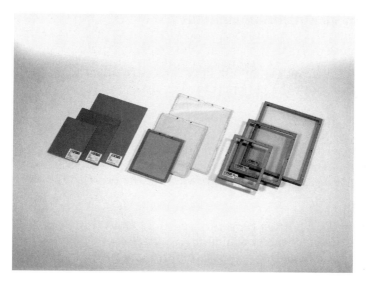

Figure 3.5. Stationary grids, covers and cassette-locating frames to allow the grid and cassette to be used as a single unit (Courtesy of Steve Dorrell, Veterinary X-Rays).

Grid ratio

This is the ratio between the height of the lead strips and the spaces in between. The larger the ratio the more efficient the grid. An average ratio in practice would be 5 : 1.

Grid factor

As the lead strips in the grid will absorb some of the primary beam, the mAs used in the exposure will have to be increased to compensate. This is known as the grid factor and will be specific to the grid used.

Film identification methods

Purpose

It is imperative that all films are permanently marked, to identify both the patient and view used.

Types

L/R marker clips
Made of stainless steel, these markers clip over the cassette to denote either the left or right view on the exposed radiograph.

Light marker
Details are written onto the record pad and transferred to the unexposed corner of film in the darkroom, leaving a permanent mark after processing has taken place.

X-Rite tape
Self-adhesive radiopaque tape on which details are recorded using a ballpoint pen. This permanently marks the exposed radiograph and can be used with personalized practice blockers recording the practice details on each radiograph.

Engraved plastic tiles
Numbers or letters are engraved into the tiles and filled with a radiopaque substance to allow permanent marking of the exposed radiograph.

Film storage envelopes
Available for tidy storage of X-ray films which ideally should be kept by the practice for a minimum of 2 years.

Positioning aids

Purpose

For the positioning of the sedated/anaesthetized animal for accurate radiographs.

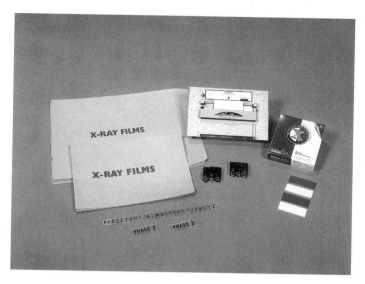

Figure 3.6. Film identification methods. Clockwise: storage envelopes, light marker, x-rite tape, plastic tiles, centre L /R clip markers (Courtesy of Steve Dorrell, Veterinary X-Rays).

Types

Ties
To secure the limbs during radiography of anaesthetized patient.

Foam wedges
Available either plain or covered in washable plastic. Wedges are radiolucent and ideal for positioning.

Sandbags
Heavier than wedges, sandbags are ideal for securing a position whilst the radiograph is being exposed.

Cradles
Radiolucent cradles or troughs are necessary for a variety of radiographic positions.

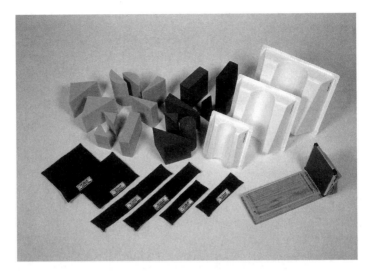

Figure 3.7. Positioning aids. Clockwise: sandbags, plain foam wedges, plastic coated foam wedges, cradles (Courtesy of Steve Dorrell, Veterinary X-Rays).

Processors

Purpose

To develop and fix the exposed film image by means of chemical reaction. This must be carried out in a darkened environment with a light filter of a specific spectrum as X-ray film is sensitive to white light.

Chemistry

Developer – converts the exposed crystals of silver bromide found on the film into minute grains of black metallic silver – forming an image. The length of time developing will take is dependent on the processor and temperature used.

Fixer – renders the image permanent, removes the unexposed silver halide crystals allowing the image to be viewed in normal light.

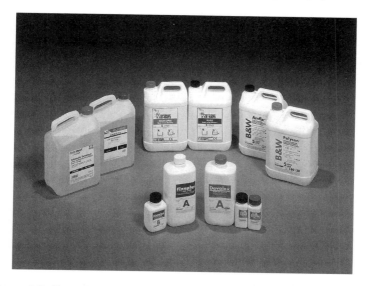

Figure 3.8. Examples of developing and fixing chemistry (Courtesy of Steve Dorrell, Veterinary X-Rays).

(a) Automatic processors

The automatic processor is made up of a light-proof cover enclosing a series of rollers through which the film passes via the developer, fixer, wash water and warm air cycles. A major advantage is that dry films of consistent quality are produced quickly, although there is some maintenance involved to keep the processor working efficiently.

Darkroom automatic processors – are loaded in the darkroom.

Daylight automatic processors – allow films to be processed without the need of a darkroom by including a light-proof attachment into which both the cassette and hands can be put to remove the film and set it onto the rollers.

(b) Manual processors

These ideally provide a facility for four of the five stages of

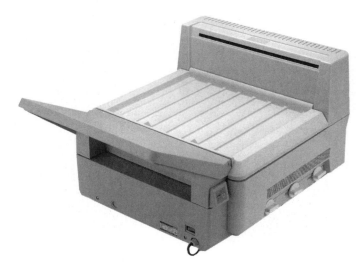

Figure 3.9. Europro darkroom automatic processor (Courtesy of Steve Dorrell, Veterinary X-Rays).

manual processing – developing, rinsing, fixing and washing. The film will still be wet after processing is completed and will need to be dried separately.

The tanks are usually suspended in a water jacket which can be thermostatically controlled.

Simpler systems may involve three tanks, developer, fixer and wash, with the developer being heated separately.

Darkroom facilities

Purpose

The darkroom should provide a suitable environment for processing exposed radiographs. It should be large enough to incorporate a wet and dry area and must be completely light proof, ideally painted in a light colour to reflect what little light is available when developing is taking place.

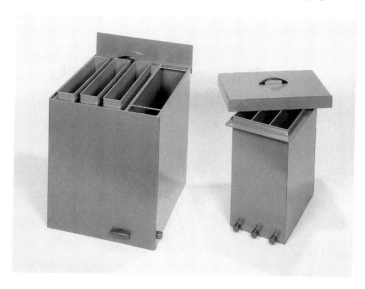

Figure 3.10. Thermostatically controlled manual processor (Courtesy of Steve Dorrell, Veterinary X-Rays).

Safelights

A box containing a low wattage bulb which has its light reduced by a safelight filter. This filters out the areas of the light spectrum to which the film is sensitive and it is important to check that the filter being used is compliant with the film being processed.

Wet bench

The area in which the processing chemicals and drying facilities for wet films may be kept in order to prevent contamination with unexposed film.

Dry bench

An area for storing film, re-loading cassettes and placing films in hangers for manual developing to take place.

Hangers

Required for manual processing. Exposed films are placed into the hanger which acts as a frame to keep the film from bending during processing and drying. Hangers come in two types – either tension clip or channel with draining racks available. Film clips are available to hang wet films from a drying line.

Thermometers and timers

Regular checking of the developer temperature prior to processing is essential for manual processing. If this is not an integral part of the machine, an alarmed timer will be required to monitor processing times.

Personal protective clothing

The operator should take great care at all times not to come into close contact with processing chemistry. Safety

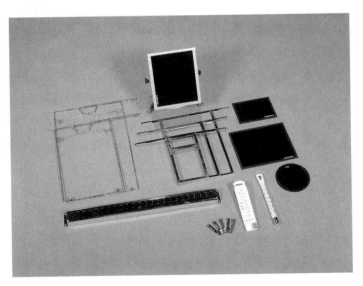

Figure 3.11. Darkroom equipment. Clockwise: clip hangers, safelight, channel hangers, safelight filters, thermometers, hanger draining rack (Courtesy of Steve Dorrell, Veterinary X-Rays).

glasses, protective aprons and gloves should be kept in the darkroom.

Recording and storage methods

Exposure chart/book

Every exposure taken in the practice should be accurately documented in an Exposure Book. Details should include patient identification, projection and exposure settings used, as well as details of the personnel and equipment (screen/film/grid combination, etc.) involved (an example is given on the next page).

Filing methods

X-Ray films should be filed in an easily accessible manner. There is no statutory obligation to keep radiographs, but the Royal College of Veterinary Surgeons (RCVS) recommends keeping them for a minimum of six years and the Veterinary Defence Society recommends keeping them for at least two years.

Ref. Number	Date	Patient/Client	Weight	Examination Area	KV/mA	Time	Comments

(Adapted from *The Exposure Book*, Veterinary X-Rays, 1998)

4
Specialized equipment

Contrast media

Purpose

To enable structures to become more apparent by either changing the radiopacity of the structure itself or by altering the structure of the tissues that surround it.

Classes

Positive
Substances of a high atomic number, therefore showing as radiopaque on the exposed film – positive contrast with other structures.

Examples:

Barium sulphate – atomic number 56. A white chalky substance available as a liquid, paste or powder to be mixed with water. Used for studies of the gastro-intestinal tract and surrounding structures. Gives excellent contrast.

Water soluble iodine compounds – atomic number 53. These are water soluble and can be injected into blood vessels to outline the urinary tract, etc. Water-soluble iodine compounds are available in many different types depending on the study they are required for.

Negative
Appear as radiolucent on the exposed film and are gases of low

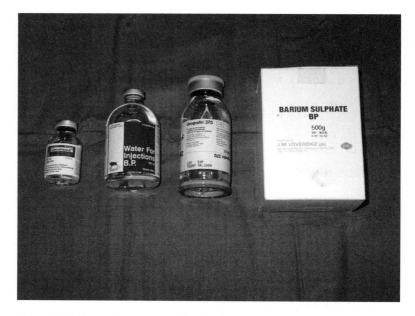

Figure 4.1. Types of contrast media. L to R: omnipaque (iodine compound used in myelography), water for injection (to dilute), urografin (iodine compound used in studies of the upper urinary system), barium sulphate.

density – negative contrast with other structures. Air is commonly used in veterinary practice.

Imaging equipment

Diagnostic ultrasound

Uses soundwaves to produce an image by converting the vibration of returning waves into electrical activity which can be converted into an image by a computer. Becoming more and more popular in practice, ultrasound studies are painless and safe to both patient and operator, and is ideal for producing 'moving' images such as cardiac function. However, the soundwaves are unable to penetrate bone or air so is of little use for the skeletal system or lung studies.

The equipment consists of a computer, a monitor and a transducer with a printer for recording images. Transducers are either 'linear' with a rectangular image, or 'sector' with a triangular image. Linear transducers require a long contact area so are more popular with rectal investigations in large animals. Sector transducers, on the other hand, are more suitable for small animal work as they require only a small contact area.

Magnetic resonance imaging (MRI)

Combining magnetism and radio energy, MRI uses a very powerful magnet as a scanner which subjects the patient to radio waves. Signals from the waves are converted into an image by a computer. Used as a referral option for diagnosis of brain disease in small animals.

Computed tomography (CT scanning)

A very detailed cross-sectional radiograph which is produced by X-ray exposure that moves along the patient showing a different 'slice' each time. Very valuable for imaging the skeletal system, CT scanning is available at referral centres and uses high levels of radiation.

Fluoroscopy

This technique is useful for evaluating gastro-intestinal anatomy and function, assisting in surgical procedures to monitor respiratory and cardiac function. Fluoroscopy is the opposite of conventional radiography, as it utilizes special screens to replace radiographic film which produce a 'positive' image rather than the usual 'negative' image seen on a conventional radiograph, i.e. the black and white areas are reversed.

The equipment used includes a screen placed above the table with the X-ray tube head under the table directed at the screen. The image on the screen is viewed through leaded glass to protect the operator from radiation.

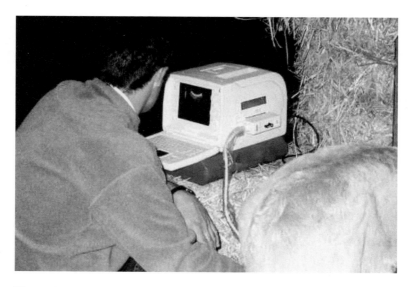

Figure 4.2. Ultrasound machine (Courtesy of BCF Technology).

Ancillary equipment

Personal protective equipment (PPE)

Purpose
To minimize the risk of radiation reaching the operator and assistants. It should be remembered that the wearing of PPE does not ensure radiation safety, and all personnel should be as far away from the primary beam as possible during exposure.

Types

- Lead aprons
- Thyroid shields
- Lead gloves and mittens
- Lead sleeves

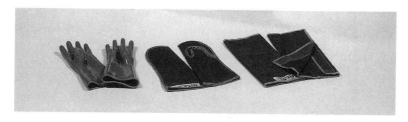

Figure 4.3. Protective gloves (Courtesy of Steve Dorrell, Veterinary X-Rays).

Basic skin preparation kit

- Electric clippers
- Disposable gloves and apron
- Surgical scrub solution, e.g. chlorhexidine
- Swabs
- Surgical spirit
- Clinical waste bin

Intravenous catheter placement kit

- Skin preparation kit
- Scalpel blade
- Heparin saline
- 2 ml syringe and appropriate needle
- Intravenous catheter
- Tape, e.g. zinc oxide tape
- Warmed fluids
- Bung and three-way tap
- Clinical waste and sharps containers

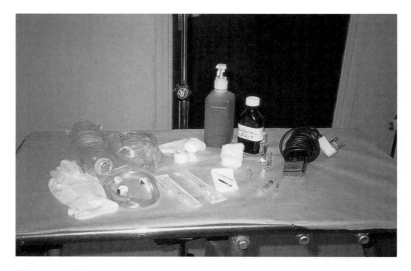

Figure 4.4. Skin preparation and intravenous catheter placement kits.

Urinary catheter placement kit

- Disposable gloves and apron
- Kidney dish
- Sterile sample pot
- Catheter
- Lubricant
- Selection of syringes
- Three-way tap
- Paper towel

5
Kits

Basic positioning kit

1   X-Ray machine – stationary, mobile or portable
2   X-Ray table – lead lined or Potter Bucky
3   X-Ray cassette with intensifying screens and film (ensure adequate size cassette chosen for area to be radiographed and sufficient number of cassettes and films available for series of exposures or complex studies)
4   Identification marker – name, rate and L/R marker
5   Grid – for tissue of 10 cm in depth or greater (optional)
6   Positioning aids – sandbags, foam wedges, ties, troughs/cradles
7   Personal protective equipment – lead aprons, gloves, screen, dosemeters

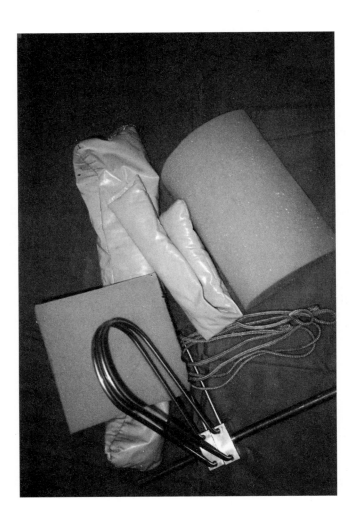

Figure 5.1. Basic positioning aids: Cradle, ties, foam wedges, sandbags.

Kits for specialized techniques

Contrast studies of the gastro-intestinal tract

Upper gastro-intestinal tract

BARIUM SWALLOW

a) *Patient preparation*

none necessary

b) *Equipment*
- General radiography preparation kit
- Barium sulphate preparation
- Catheter tip syringe (optional)
- Canned pet food (optional)
- Absorbent material
- Gloves and apron

NB: Care must be exercised during administration of barium to avoid any spillage onto radiographic equipment, patient or personnel.

BARIUM STUDY

a) *Patient preparation*
- Fast for 12–24 hours
- Enema 2–4 hours prior to procedure (optional)
- Mild sedation (optional)

b) *Equipment*
- General radiography preparation kit
- Barium sulphate preparation
- Orogastric tube (optional)
- Catheter tip syringe
- Absorbent material
- Gloves and aprons

NB: Care must be exercised during administration of barium to avoid any spillage onto radiographic equipment, patient or personnel.

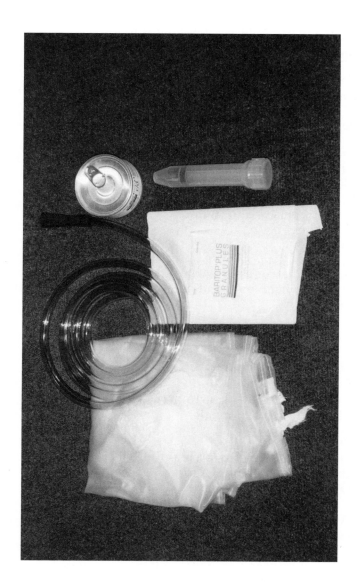

Figure 5.2. Barium studies kit. L to R: disposable gloves and apron, orogastric tube, barium sulphate preparation, paper towel, canned food, syringe.

Lower gastro-intestinal tract

BARIUM ENEMA

a) *Patient preparation*
- Low residue diet 48 hours prior to study
- Enema 12 hours in advance until clear

b) *Equipment*
- General radiography preparation kit
- Barium sulphate liquid preparation
- Foley/balloon tip catheter
- Catheter tip syringe
- Lubricant
- Forceps to clamp catheter
- Gloves and aprons

NB: Care must be exercised to avoid barium spillage on radiographic equipment, patient and personnel.

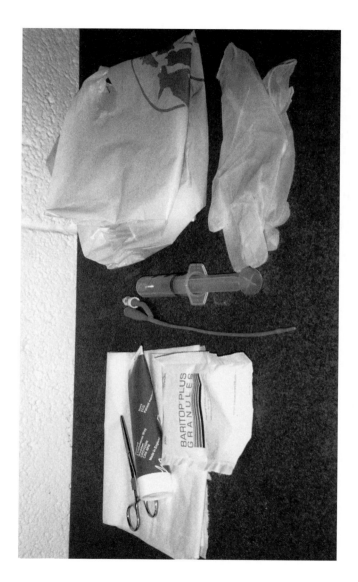

Figure 5.3. Barium enema kit. L to R: paper towel, forceps, lubricant, barium preparation, Foley catheter, catheter tip syringe, disposable gloves and apron.

Contrast studies of the urinary system

Upper urinary system

EXCRETION UROGRAPHY/INTRAVENOUS UROGRAM OR PYELOGRAM

a) *Patient preparation*
- Fast 12–24 hours prior to study
- Cleansing enema 4 hours prior to study
- Sedation or general anaesthesia (optional)

b) *Equipment*
- General radiography preparation equipment
- Water soluble iodinated compound
- Intravenous placement kit
- Syringe for contrast agent

NB: Care must be exercised to avoid spillage of contrast agent on radiographic equipment, patient or personnel.

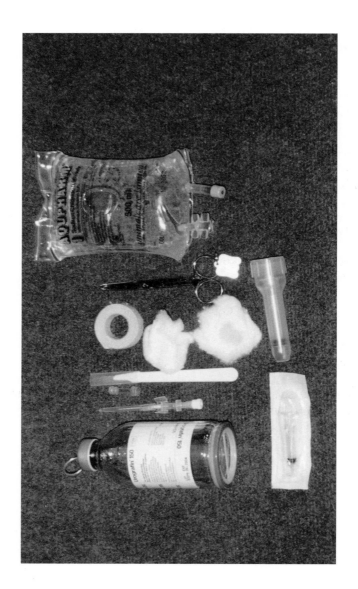

Figure 5.4. Excretion urography kit. L to R: contrast media, syringe, IV placement kit.

Lower urinary system

CYSTOGRAPHY (± RETROGRADE URETHROGRAM OR VAGINOGRAM)

a) *Patient preparation*
   - Fast 12–24 hours
   - Cleansing enema 4 hours prior to study

b) *Equipment – negative contrast cystogram* (Pneumocystogram)
   - General radiography preparation kit
   - Speculum
   - Urinary catheter
   - Syringes 3 ml–60 ml selection
   - Lubricant
   - Three-way tap
   - Kidney dish
   - Sterile universal container
   - Gloves and apron

c) *Equipment – double contrast and positive contrast cystogram*
   - As above part b)
   - Water soluble iodinated compound (30% dilution)

NB: Care must be exercised to avoid spillage of contrast agent on radiographic equipment, patient or personnel.

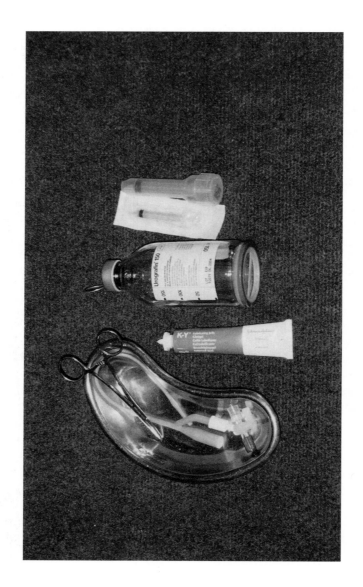

Figure 5.5. Cystography kit. L to R: kidney dish, three-way tap, catheter, forceps, lubricant, contrast media, syringes. A vaginal speculum, a sterile sample pot and a disposable apron and gloves will also be required.

Additional techniques

MYELOGRAPHY

a) *Patient preparation*
   - Fast 12–24 hours
   - General anaesthesia

b) *Equipment*
   - General radiography preparation kit
   - Skin preparation kit
   - Marker pen with area identified – cisternal or lumbar puncture
   - Spinal needle
   - Low osmolar, non ionic water soluble iodinated compound
   - Sterile sample pot
   - Syringes 2–10 ml selection
   - Sandbags and foam wedges to raise patient's head
   - Gloves and apron

NB: Safety point
Ensure kennel prepared for recovery with area to keep patient's head raised. Patient should be observed continuously until able to maintain sternal recumbancy.

Care must be exercised to avoid spillage of contrast agent on radiographic equipment, patient or personnel.

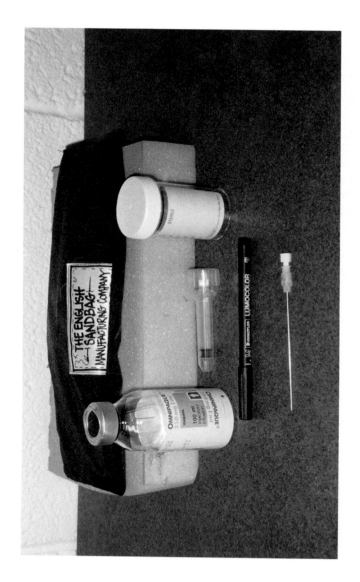

Figure 5.6. Myelography kit. L to R: foam wedge and sandbag, contrast agent, marker pen, spinal needle, syringe, sterile sample pot.

ANGIOGRAPHY, ARTHOGRAPHY, CARDIOGRAPHY, VENOGRAPHY

a) *Patient preparation*

- Sedation or general anaesthetic (optional)
- Prepare skin relevant to area of study

b) *Equipment*

- General radiography preparation kit
- Skin preparation kit
- Intravenous kit and appropriate sized catheter
- Water soluble iodinated compound
- Nitrous oxide or air for arthrogram (optional)
- Waterproof marker pen
- Sterile sample pot
- Gloves and apron

NB: Care must be exercised to avoid spillage of contrast agent on radiography equipment, patient or personnel.

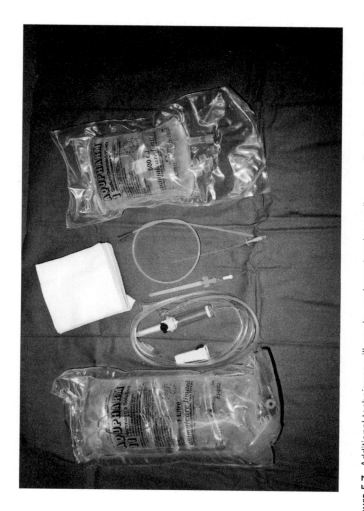

Figure 5.7. Additional techniques will require equipment such as saline as well as the appropriate contrast media.

6
Reference images of specialized techniques

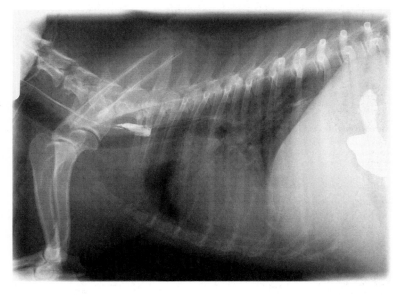

Barium swallow. Post barium with meat. There is gas in the cervical oesophagus. A bolus of barium/meat is rostral to the heart base and there is a narrowed area over the heart base. Diagnosis of oesophageal stricture (Courtesy of Queens Veterinary School Hospital, University of Cambridge).

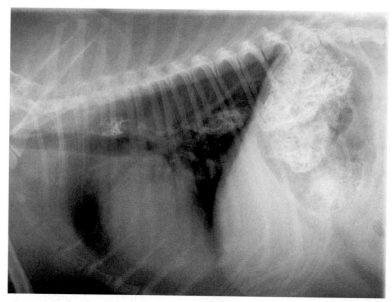

Barium swallow. There is some barium retained just caudal to the thoracic inlet in the oesophagus suggesting poor motility. Diagnosis of mega colon from subsequent radiographs (Courtesy of Queens Veterinary School Hospital, University of Cambridge).

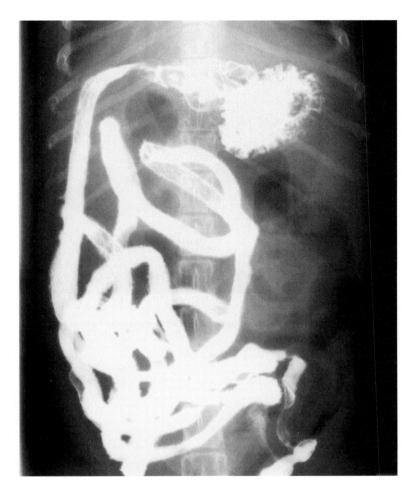

Barium study. Upper gastrointestinal tract. Ventral dorsal view. Thirty minutes post barium. Diagnosis: mild gastritis (Courtesy of Queens Veterinary School Hospital, University of Cambridge).

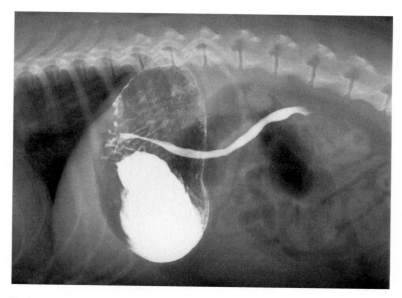

Barium study. Upper gastrointestinal tract. Lateral view. Diagnosis: mild gastritis (Courtesy of Queens Veterinary School Hospital, University of Cambridge).

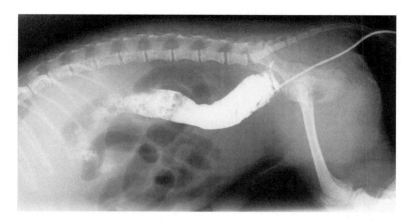

Barium enema. The outline of the Foley catheter can be seen. No diagnosis due to the presence of faecal material (Courtesy of Queens Veterinary School Hospital, University of Cambridge).

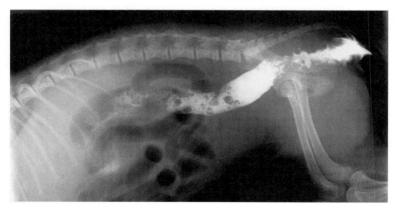

Barium enema. No diagnosis due to the presence of faecal material (Courtesy of Queens Veterinary School Hospital, University of Cambridge).

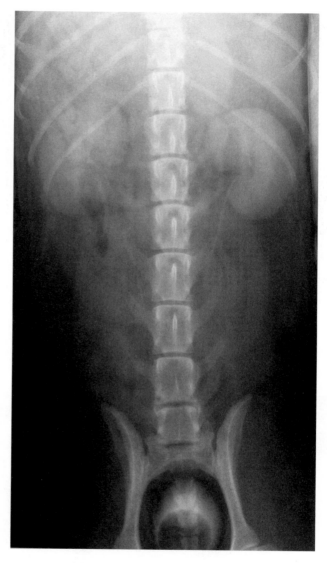

Intravenous urethrogram. Ventral dorsal view. IVU normal. Diagnosis of vestibulovaginal stricture from subsequent radiographs (Courtesy of Queens Veterinary School Hospital, University of Cambridge).

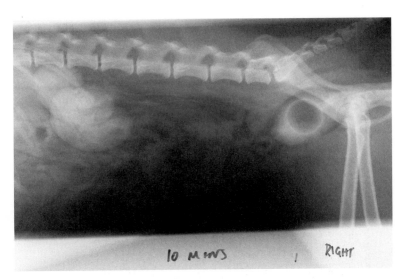

Intravenous urethrogram. Lateral view. IVN normal. Diagnosis of vestibulovaginal stricture from subsequent radiographs (Courtesy of Queens Veterinary School Hospital, University of Cambridge).

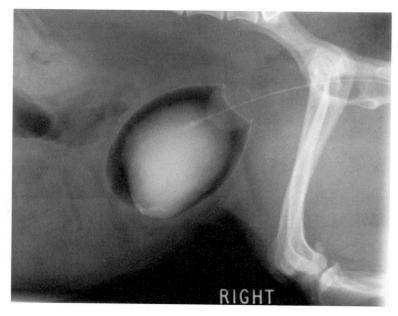

Double contrast cystogram. Patient presented with persistent haematuria.
There is marked thickening of the bladder wall consistent with chronic cystitis
(Courtesy of Queens Veterinary School Hospital, University of Cambridge).

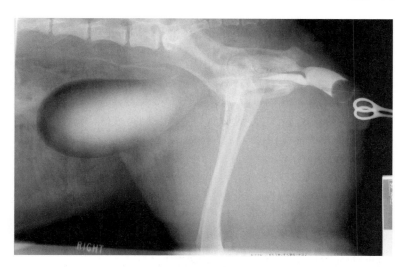

Vaginourethrogram. Diagnosis: vestibulovaginal syndrome (Courtesy of Queens Veterinary School Hospital, University of Cambridge).

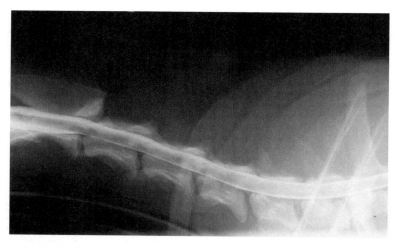

Cervical myelogram. Normal (Courtesy of Queens Veterinary School Hospital, University of Cambridge).

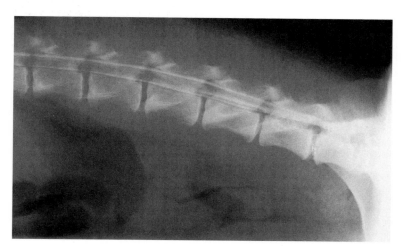

Lumbar myelogram. Narrowing of intervertebral disc space T12–13 and T13–L1 and dorsal deviation of ventral column over intravertebral disc space T12–13 (Courtesy of Queens Veterinary School Hospital, University of Cambridge).

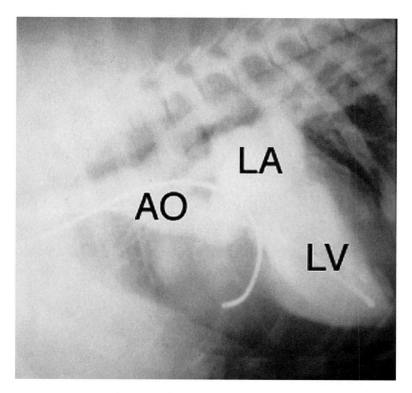

Cardiogram. LA = left atrium; LV = left ventricle; AO = aorta.

Diagnosis: sub aortic stenosis in a Rottweiler (Courtesy of Queens Veterinary School Hospital, University of Cambridge).

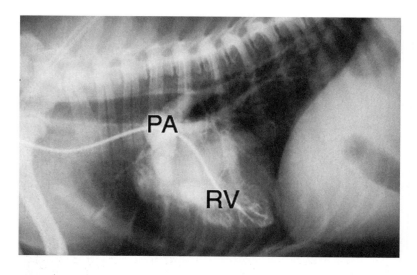

Cardiogram. RV = right ventricle; PA = pulmonary artery.

Diagnosis: pulmonic stenosis in a West Highland White Terrier (Courtesy of Queens Veterinary School Hospital, University of Cambridge).

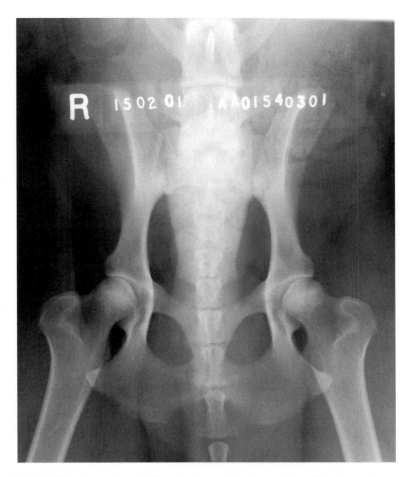

British Veterinary Association hip dysplasia scheme X-ray (Courtesy of Queens Veterinary School Hospital, University of Cambridge).

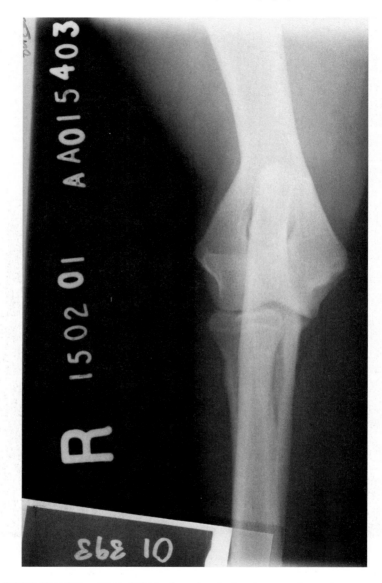

British Veterinary Association elbow dysplasia scheme radiograph
(Courtesy of Queens Veterinary School Hospital, University of Cambridge).

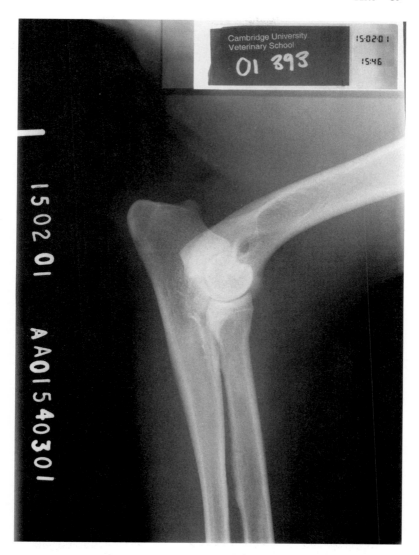

British Veterinary Association elbow dysplasia scheme radiograph
(Courtesy of Queens Veterinary School Hospital, University of Cambridge).

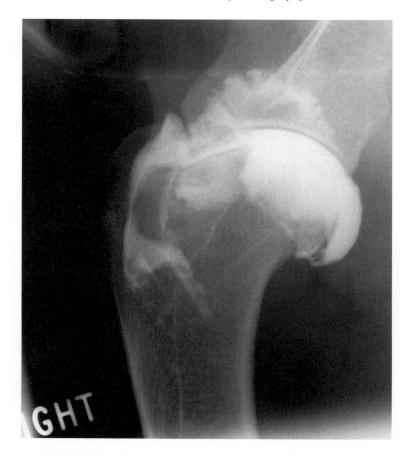

Shoulder arthrogram. There is an irregularity of contrast line around the bicipital tendon. Diagnosis: bicipital tendonitis (Courtesy of Queens Veterinary School Hospital, University of Cambridge).

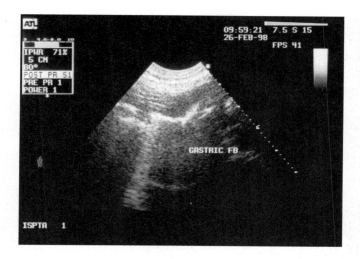

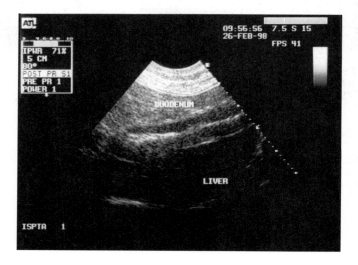

Ultrasound (Courtesy of Queens Veterinary School Hospital, University of Cambridge).

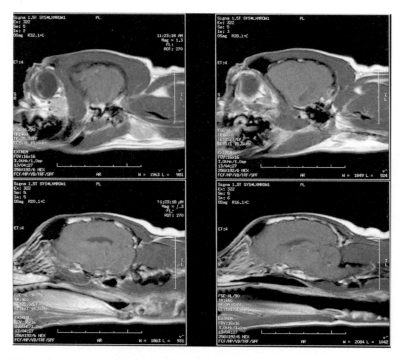

Magnetic Resonance Image. The crossbreed was presented with neurological signs but no diagnosis was made (Courtesy of Queens Veterinary School Hospital, University of Cambridge).

7
Self-assessment

Across
1. X-Ray of the bladder
3. Measure of current
6. Filters out light
7. Absorbs scatter
8. X-Ray of a joint
9. Reflection of waves

Down
1. Reduction of beam
2. Renders permanent
4. Sensitive crystal
5. Contains screens

(*Answers on Page 67*)

How well do you score on radiography?

Multiple choice

1. A **lateromedial** projection refers to the X-ray beam:

    (a) entering the limb through the medial side and exiting from the lateral side
    (b) entering the limb through the lateral side and exiting from the medial side
    (c) being directed towards the left side of the body and emerging on the right
    (d) being directed towards the right side of the body and emerging on the left

2. **Arthrography** is a radiographic study of the:

    (a) heart
    (b) stomach
    (c) kidney
    (d) joint

3. **Cystography** is a radiographic study of the:

    (a) spinal cord
    (b) kidneys
    (c) bladder
    (d) bile duct

4. The term **Palmar** refers to the:

    (a) caudal aspect of the forelimb distal to the carpus joint
    (b) cranial aspect of the forelimb distal to the carpus joint
    (c) caudal aspect of the forelimb distal to the tarsus joint
    (d) cranial aspect of the forelimb distal to the tarsus joint

5. The definition of **kilovoltage** (Kv) is the:

   (a) current of X-rays
   (b) penetrating power of X-rays
   (c) quality of X-rays
   (d) timing of X-rays

6. **Barium sulphate** is an example of a:

   (a) negative insoluble contrast agent
   (b) negative soluble contrast agent
   (c) positive insoluble contrast agent
   (d) positive soluble contrast agent

7. The person responsible for drawing up the **Local Rules and System of Work** for radiography procedures is the:

   (a) Practice Principal
   (b) Health and Safety Executive
   (c) Radiation Protection Adviser
   (d) Radiation Protection Supervisor

8. The **Grid Factor** relates to the amount by which the:

   (a) mAs must be increased
   (b) mAs must be decreased
   (c) kV must be increased
   (d) kV must be decreased

9. The film and screen combination that provides the **best** detail is:

   (a) slow film/slow screen
   (b) slow film/fast screen
   (c) fast film/slow screen
   (d) fast film/fast screen

10. A Potter Bucky diaphragm is an example of a:

    (a) pseudofocused grid
    (b) moving grid
    (c) focused grid
    (d) stationary grid

11. Processed radiographs should **ideally** be stored for a minimum of:

    (a) one year
    (b) two years
    (c) five years
    (d) ten years

12. The veterinary association responsible for providing the **Hip Dysplasia** scoring scheme is:

    (a) BVHA
    (b) BVA
    (c) BVNA
    (d) BSAVA

13. The **minimum** distance for personnel to be near the primary beam is:

    (a) 0.5 metres
    (b) 1 metre
    (c) 1.5 metres
    (d) 2 metres

14. Diagnostic ultrasound produces an imagine by means of:

    (a) soundwaves
    (b) fluoroscopy
    (c) magnetic forces
    (d) radiation

15. An **intravenous urogram** is a contrast study of the:

    (a) circulatory system
    (b) reproductive system
    (c) neurological system
    (d) urinary system

Answer key

						¹C	Y	S	T	O	G	R	A	M
				²F		O								
			³M	I	L	L	I	A	M	P	E	⁴R	E	
		⁵C		X		L						A		
	⁶S	A	F	E	L	I	G	H	T		⁷G	R	I	D
		S		R		M						E		
		S				A						E		
		E		⁸A	R	T	H	R	O	G	R	A	M	
		T				I						R		
⁹U	L	T	R	A	S	O	U	N	D			T		
		E				N						H		

Multiple choice

1	b	6	d	11	b
2	d	7	c	12	b
3	c	8	a	13	d
4	a	9	a	14	a
5	b	10	b	15	d

Selected reading

Veterinary Nursing, 2nd edition, 1999, Lane & Cooper. Butterworth-Heinemann, ISBN 0-7506-3999-7

Principles of Veterinary Radiography, 2nd edition, 1975, Douglas & Williamson. Baillière, ISBN 0-7020-0381-6

Manual of Radiography & Radiology in Small Animal Practice, R. Lee, 1990, BSAVA Publication, ISBN 0-905214-102

Radiography in Veterinary Technology, 2nd edition, 1998, Lisa M. Lavin. WB Saunders, ISBN 0-7216-7552-2

Index

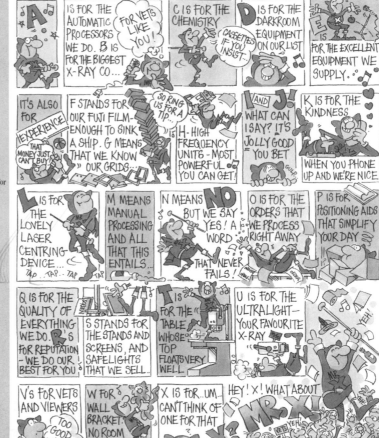
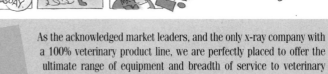
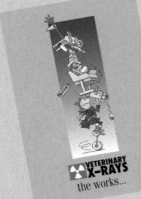
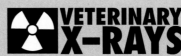